Disclaimer:

The information in this book is not intended as a substitute for the advice of trained medical or mental health professionals. The reader should regularly consult a physician, therapist or counselor in matters relating to his/ her physical or mental health and particularly with respect to any symptoms that may require diagnosis or medical attention. In the event you use any of the information in this book, the author and the publisher assume no responsibility for your actions.

Table of Contents:

Acknowledgements

I would like to thank the people at selfpublishing-school, my friends and my family who helped with everything surrounding this book. A special thanks to Beeldenstorm.nl for their great advice, Koen Bouman for the filming and editing, my girlfriend for always supporting me and to my mother, who was a big inspiration for this book.

Introduction:

In today's world, starting a new diet is as common as buying new clothes. The difference is, when you start a diet, some people encourage you, while others give you the same patronizing look they would give to a dog when it tries to catch its own tail. In 2014, 39% of adults worldwide were overweight. As a species, we have come to an embarrassing point. More people in the world die from complications of being overweight and obese than from those of being underweight[1].

In general, we know what to do about being overweight, so why don't we all do it? Most overweight people have started diets at some point, but very few make it to the lean finish line. I'm sure I've sparked a few critics by now who say, 'Well my friend lost (insert high number) of weight in (insert low number) of days'. That's very possible; I once lost 10 pounds in 3 days as an experiment, but it's one of the worst things you can do if you want to lose weight permanently. There is a very high chance that one year later, that person will be right back where he or she started, or maybe even heavier. This book will guide you through the horrendously confusing world of dieting and show you how you can attack weight loss with brains and brawn. I'll show how you can enjoy food, lose weight and not feel like killing yourself while doing it.

I've always been intrigued by the way our bodies work. My quest for health started when I was around 14. I experimented on myself with different eating styles: paleo, intermittent fasting, high carb, low carb, no carb, etc. My interest in food and health made me choose to study Health and Nutrition at Wageningen University, one of the top universities for everything nutrition related.

This book is meant to counteract the scams, lies, misinformation and confusion I have found. Before I learned about nutrition and health, I was confused because of the many misleading opinions and 'facts' that floated around the internet. The media also does its fair share to add to the confusion.

Just recently, a study found that people who eat more processed meat have a 6% chance of getting colorectal cancer, compared to 5% for people who eat less processed meat[2]. A few days later the news was filled with headlines like: 'Bacon is more dangerous than asbestos', '20x higher chance of cancer when you eat processed meat', and my personal favourite: 'Can we eat anything without dying?' If you do, you'll be the first.

Newspapers, sites, and blogs make money by attracting you to read or watch their stories, so they sensationalise everything that is remotely interesting. The superfood hype is also a recent example. People started eating overpriced bird seed and spent ridiculous amounts of money on some 'all curing' berries. I understand that food is a tricky subject to tackle. Because food is something with which we all have experience, it's easy to form an opinion on it. That said, allow me to lift the curtain and let you into the world of science-based, healthy eating.

My goal is not just to help you lose weight. I want - and I assume you do as well - to keep the fat off permanently. This book will show you how most people approach dieting ineffectively, setting themselves up to fail. Then we'll delve into a mini masterclass on nutrition. This will teach you everything you need to know to avoid being fooled by marketing gimmicks, and it will give you the proper ammo to shoot down any food related nonsense that comes up at your next dinner party.

If you apply the knowledge from this book, you will lose weight. I'll go even further and say that with the right mindset, this book will be your guide to a diet-free life. For me this has meant not having to worry about my weight, eating delicious food, and enjoying great health, and now I have the opportunity to share what I've learned and help you to achieve the same things.

I must warn you, just reading this book will not get you anywhere. You may learn a thing or two about nutrition, which in itself is valuable, but then you're missing the point of this book. I challenge you to make a change and commit to your health. Too many people wait for things to happen, and as a result they don't achieve what they set out to do. This book has the potential to change your life, but I cannot be there to hold your hand. Therefore I ask you to commit to this journey and hold yourself to a high standard. People who wait get left out. Care enough about your health to make a change and master this part of your life.

1. Why Do People Get Fat?

Three main factors determine if a person gets fat or not. We'll start very small and work our way up to bigger things.

Genetics determine how everything in our bodies is designed. You can change very little about this, like the fact that some people have blue eyes and others have brown ones. Genetics also plays a major role in fat loss, because some people are just more inclined to gain fat. This is caused by abnormal levels of ghrelin, one of the hunger hormones[3]. Your genes also determine where your body prefers to store fat. Some people store a lot of fat on their legs, while others store more fat around their love handles. Just because you may be more inclined to gain weight than others, that does not mean your situation is hopeless by any means. Anyone can lose weight, even if you have 'fat genes'.

Genes can hardly be changed once you have them, but not all of your genes are active all the time. They can be turned on or off like a light switch. The field that studies this process is called epigenetics. Epigenetics is a relatively new field of science, but it's a very cool one. There is still much research to be done, but some say that epigenetics has the potential to explain aging, disease, the origin of cancer, heart disease and mental illness. There are signs that the food we eat influences which of our genes can be passed on. This means your food choices could influence your offspring[4].

It is said that we are the products of our environments, and in many ways this is true. Your environment consists of everything that influences you, like your friends, family, the country you live in, your culture, movies, music, and books. All these things combined essentially shape who you are. More importantly for the subject of weight loss, they determine if you get fat. If your parents are fat because of their bad eating habits and you are raised with those same habits and similar genes, chances are that you will be fat as an adult, too. The worst part is that many people simply do not know any better, or they do but they don't know where to start. Little kids have nothing to say about the foods their parents serve them. Learning how to eat healthy not only helps yourself, but it also helps future generations.

2. Why Diets Fail

Meet Emma. Emma is a mother of three, and her weight has always been a struggle since life overwhelmed her with work, kids to raise, a relationship, and a social life to maintain. She is not one to give up easily, though, and she has tried lots of things to lose weight. But no matter what type of diet she tries, they all seem to fail. Some diets cause her to lose weight very quickly the first few days or weeks, but eventually the weight loss seems to stall and her motivation drops.

When the diets end she is semi happy with the result. Sure, the process wasn't fun, but at least she fits in her jeans again. After the diet, life kicks in again. She gets stressed out over work, and the kids hit puberty. Slowly but surely the weight starts to creep on again. When she realizes she is heavier now than before she started the diet, her spirit drops like sack of potatoes. All the hard work she'd put in was for nothing. She blames herself for not being 'strong' enough, and she decides to start even crazier diets.

'Emma' is an example of the stories I've heard and read over the last few years from people who have been let down by diets. Most of the popular diets today (Atkins, paleo, etc.) are pretty effective at reducing your weight while you're on the diet, but that is also their greatest limitation. They are effective while you are on the diet, not once you are finished. My goal is to break the 'diet cycle' of weight loss, regain, pain and repeat.

Weight loss happens when a person burns more calories (kcal) than he or she consumes. The concept of calories isn't just thrown around to sell diets; it's a unit to measure the energy stored in food. Your body is a busy machine, and all kinds of processes require energy: your brain, your muscles when you move, repairing damage, and millions of other processes.

The average female needs 2000kcal per day. So if a woman eats 1800kcal on a particular day, her body has to use some of its stored energy (like body fat) to get the missing 200kcal. This is how you lose weight: you eat less than you burn. It's called a calorie deficit. Sounds simple enough, right? For gaining weight, it's the exact opposite, you eat more than your body burns, and your body stores the remainder for later. This is called a calorie surplus.

This method of storing excess body fat was quite useful in 10000 BC. Slaying a mammoth meant there was enough food for a while, so our bodies stored the excess energy to provide a buffer for when scarcer times arrived. Our bodies are particularly interested in fat-rich and sugar-rich foods because they provide a nice kcal punch, and that's what we used to need to survive. We like to think we have evolved or grown as a species, and indeed we have done some amazing things like make people fly, cure a ton of diseases and invent the internet. But deep down, despite all the amazing progress, we are physiologically still the same mammoth slaying people with the same nutritional desires.

Fast forward to 2015. Kcal-dense foods are now everywhere, and instead of having to get out and get our food by hunting, you can hunt down the nearest pizza place on the internet. You could eat a different meal every day for weeks without even having to leave the house. Your body doesn't care that you don't want to be overweight; it just wants to survive. If you're hungry and you see a delicious cheeseburger, your body sends out some pretty convincing signals that you have to eat that cheeseburger. It's the way we are designed, and it's not going to change any time soon.

This major shift from scarcity to abundance is one of the main reasons many people today are overweight. We have only really had an overflow of food for the past few decades, but our bodies still work through the same survival mechanisms as 10000 years ago.
Another big reason is the increasing availability of fat and sugar-rich foods. To make matters even worse, we are bombarded with some pretty amazing advertising by companies like Coca Cola and McDonald's. I personally don't care much for their products, but their marketing departments are amazing. Credit where credit is due. This overflow of stimuli combined with the increasing access to calorie-rich foods is a major issue.

You must understand that this does not mean that all hope is lost, but I think it's important to understand what is happening inside and around you when it comes to food. The famous 12-step plan from Alcoholics Anonymous tells you to start with the first step: acknowledging that you have a problem. To change weight, it is crucial to understand the mismatch between today's environment and the way our bodies are designed.

Willpower

When people are asked why they failed a diet (or, I should say, the diet failed them), one of the most prominent answers is that they didn't have enough self discipline or willpower. The American Psychological Association describes willpower as follows[5]:

'At its essence, willpower is the ability to resist short-term temptations in order to meet long-term goals.'

Willpower is a tricky fellow when it comes to dieting. In their book *Willpower, Rediscovering the Greatest Human Strength*[6], Roy Baumeister and John Tierney say that humans can perform extraordinary acts of will in certain circumstances, but go on to say that dieting is a special case. They call it the 'Oprah paradox', named after one of the most successful people on the planet, Oprah Winfrey. Despite having achieved incredible business success, which requires an enormous amount of willpower, she still seems to have trouble with her weight.

Oprah has access to an incredible team of personal trainers, chefs, coaches and support, but she still regains weight each and every time. Willpower is useful in every day life, but dieting has some special hidden traps. Baumeister, in cooperation with Dutch scientists, found that people with a high amount of willpower have more success in their business lives, at school and in their relationships, but they only have a very small advantage when in comes to losing weight long term[7].

One of the big drawbacks of relying on willpower is that it is depletable. Nobel prize winner Daniel Kahneman describes it beautifully in his book *Thinking, Fast and Slow*[8]. He describes our minds as divided into two systems (some neuroscientists will have taken that literally and started sending out hate mail to Mr. Kahneman, but the metaphor works for explaining behaviour). The fast system is our automatic pilot. We use this system most of the time because it takes little effort to use, and it gives us decent results most of the time. The fast system is responsible for all tasks that require little mental effort and can be done on auto pilot, like walking, driving a familiar route, some regular chitchat with a colleague, or brushing our teeth. The slow system kicks in when mental effort is required, like when we have to solve puzzles, answer hard questions, or take tests.

Humans are the only species that is self aware, and we have the amazing capability to use our slow systems to consciously ignore the fast system's programming and make better choices. This is why we are able to make decisions focused on long-term gain instead of just focusing on short-term satisfaction. For example, when you decide to eat a home cooked meal instead of ordering a pizza. Your fast system would love the instant gratification it gets from all those delicious calories in that pizza, but you are better off long term if you decide to eat the healthier meal.

Baumeister's research shows that the effort involved in self control or willpower is tiring. It takes effort to override your fast system. If you exert mental effort at a task and shortly thereafter a second task arises, you are less capable of providing the same mental effort. Baumeister also found that all mentally demanding tasks seem to draw from the same pool of mental energy: glucose. The nervous system is the highest comsumer of glucose in our bodies.

Baumeister found that when our brains run out of glucose, our willpower is also gone. The process of our brains spending energy to make conscious decisions is known as *ego depletion* or *decision fatigue*. What's interesting is that people's ability to override the fast system and make intelligent decisions increases once they have consumed glucose. Practical application: This does not mean you should slam down glucose each time you have to make a decision. A good meal keeps your glucose levels stable for quite some time.

What ego depletion means in practice is that when you have spent your brain power on a difficult task, the coming tasks have to be done with a lower amount of willpower. Let's say you're driving home from work after a long day and you're feeling hungry. You've exhausted your mind with all kinds of tasks throughout the day, and now the choice has to be made what you are going to eat for dinner. As you're driving home you see a giant, beautiful, yellow 'M' at the side of the road. Your body is naturally more inclined toward choosing the fatty and sugary foods (this is coming from the automatic fast brain), and now effort has to be generated to override the fast system and choose something more nutritious using your active slow brain.

Unfortunately your brain is out of glucose from the work you've done, and you can't muster up the energy to make the better choice. You let your auto pilot kick in, and you end up with greasy hands and a mixed feeling of satisfaction and guilt. When your willpower is low, your fast system makes all the food choices. This means that the food you eat is habitual and automatic instead of a real choice.

Jonathan Haidt, in his book *The Happiness Hypothesis*[9] describes the fast system as the elephant and the slow system as the rider. Although the rider is 'in control', the elephant is much stronger than the rider. The rider cannot force the elephant to go anywhere. The elephant has to be persuaded to do so. Haidt says that learning how to train the elephant is the secret to self-improvement. We'll discover how to do this in the next chapter.

The downfall of restrictive dieting

The best way to assure someone will do something is to tell him he is not allowed to do it. This is why restrictive dieting fails. Psychologist Daniel Wegner showed this in his famous 'white bear experiments'. Volunteers were asked not to think of a white bear, and sure enough, after a few seconds or minutes, a polar bear popped up[10].

 Our affection for polar bears is fairly limited most of the time, so imagine how much your mind would struggle with something as attractive as delicious food. If a diet dictates that you cannot eat pizza for the coming weeks, you can be sure you'll want pizza soon, even if you wouldn't have wanted it without the diet.

Restriction in action

An interesting study was done to study the effects of a preload (a meal before the main experiment) on the intake of cookies and crackers[11].

The researchers asked three groups of people to judge some cookies and crackers. They all hadn't eaten for a while before the experiment (this was a requirement), so all three groups were hungry. One group got a small milkshake (a small preload) to kill the hunger a little bit, another group got nothing, and the last group got two enormous milkshakes (a big preload), with enough kcals to satiate the average person. Within each of these groups were dieters and non-dieters.

The actual aim of the experiment was to see how many crackers and cookies each group would eat. The participants weren't told this in advance, because if you tell people you're going to measure how much they eat, you all of a sudden get way more socially desirable results. The results for people who weren't on a diet were what you'd expect. The group that had two massive milkshakes just nibbled the cookies and crackers and ate only a little. The group that got the tiny milkshake ate a little more, and the group that ate nothing in advance ate the most of the crackers and cookies.

The results for the dieters were the exact opposite. The dieters in the group who got the two massive shakes actually ate more cookies than the group that hadn't had any food in advance.

This is called *counterregulatory eating*, or as I like to call it, 'The f*ck it effect'. People on diets usually set a certain amount of calories as the limit for that day, and they hold on to it with everything they've got. In the experiment, the two milkshakes put most dieters over their self-set daily max of calories, and what happens after is the bad part. Once their only real line has been crossed (be it in the name of science), they say 'f*ck it' and stop caring about their diets at all. They view that entire day as lost, because they have already failed in their minds. Most of the damage is actually done after they decide the day is lost, because there are no more boundaries left to cross, and everything in sight is fair game.

A follow-up study revealed a similar finding. Again, dieters and non-dieters were asked to come to the lab and not to eat in advance. Some dieters got an amount of food that put them over their daily allowances. After that, all the participants got a sandwich that was cut into four pieces. After they ate as much as they liked, everybody was unexpectedly asked how many sandwich pieces they had eaten. This isn't a hard question by any standard - they had just finished them. Most of the people could fairly accurately recall how many pieces they had eaten. There was one group, however, that failed to accurately recall how many pieces they ate: the dieters that had already surpassed their limits. As soon as they had mentally quit their diets for the day, they stopped noticing how much they ate for the rest of the experiment[12].

Note: Some lucky people lose weight on any diet, and they keep the weight off for a long period of time. Unfortunately this group is small, and you should not feel discouraged. We're here to create a smart and steady plan to lose weight that can work for the majority of people, not just a lucky few.

Chapter summary:

- Losing weight is done with a calorie deficit, gaining weight with a surplus.
- Our bodies are still the same as 10000 years ago. This creates a mismatch with today's food-rich environment.
- Your mind has two systems: the slow system and the fast system. The ability to override the fast system is limited. Willpower depletes with each choice, so spend it wisely.
- Restricting backfires.

3. What We Should Change: Habits

'Chains of habit are too light to be felt until they are too
heavy to be broken.'
-Warren Buffett

You already know your brain likes to operate on its fast
and automatic mode to save energy. This can be a
downside, but it can also be part of a strategy to turn
things around. Breaking habits can be difficult, but once
a new habit has been formed, it doesn't take much effort
to maintain it and perform the new behaviour. The
elephant doesn't have to be forced to do something it
doesn't want to.

Here are several steps to go from an old destructive
habit to forming a newer, better one. The first focus has
to be on identifying why you perform certain
behaviours.

Most habits have more than one facet. You may think
you do things for a certain reason, but unconsciously
you might have a very different motivator. It is very
important to realize why you do some things the way
you do. Once you find out what drives the behaviour,
try to experiment with different solutions to see what
really satisfies the need related to the behaviour. You'll
see an example of this down below. Spoiler: it involves
cookies.

Breaking habits

'Habit is habit, and not to be flung out of the window, but coaxed downstairs a step at a time.'
-Mark Twain

Habits can be tough to break. A 2009 study found that it takes around 66 days to break an old habit and form a new one[13]. Charles Duhigg, author of *The Power of Habit*[14], suggests there are three steps to forming a habit:

1) The trigger that tells your brain to let a certain behaviour unfold
2) The habit itself, or the associated routine
3) The reward, something that your brain likes to help it remember the habit loop

For example, the habit of smoking goes like this: first, something triggers the behaviour. A cool relative or friend offers you a cigarette. Second, the habit of smoking and third the reward of nicotine. The habit loop is now in place, and it just requires repetition to engrain.

The more engrained or automatic the habit becomes, the less energy your brain has to spend on performing the behaviour. It has become natural.

Breaking a habit therefore requires a lot of mental effort.

The basis of breaking a habit can be described as follows:

1) Recognize the behaviour.
2) Find the triggers or cues that make you perform the behaviour.
3) Remove those triggers and cues as much as possible.
4) Replace the old habit with a better, more helpful one.

Charles Duhigg talks about his own struggles with weight loss after he had gained 8.7 pounds by eating cookies each day at the office. He wondered why this was the case. He considered himself to be a successful guy. He had even just won a Pulitzer Prize, but he wasn't able to resist a few simple cookies? He found out by monitoring himself that he got the urge for a cookie each day at 15:30. His normal routine was to leave his desk, go buy a cookie, and then chat with colleagues for a bit. He decided to do some experimentation. He wanted to find out if it was the actual cookie he was craving, or if something else was giving him a reward, with the cookie just being a part of a routine.

First he tried to get up from his desk at 15:30 and walk around the block to see if it was just some activity he was craving. The second day he went down to the cafeteria, bought a candy bar instead of a cookie and went straight up to his desk to eat it, instead of talking to his colleagues. The third day he left his again at 15:30, but instead of buying anything, he just chatted with his colleagues for a few minutes and then went back to work. He found out that he was the happiest when he ate no cookie and just socialized with his colleagues for a while. He found out what it was that gave him the reward, and since then he has lost 12 pounds.

Let's take another look at the example from Chapter 1, in which you were on your way home from work exhausted and had to resist the urge to splurge at your local fast food chain. With your willpower zapped from the work you'd done and the amazing advertisements by the fast food chains, you never really stood a chance. (Seriously, those guys know how to market their stuff.) In this case, it is mostly about removing the triggers that cause you to perform the behaviour.

The triggers here are the advertisements and the feeling of hunger combined with low willpower. To avoid the advertisements, you could take another route back from work where you know you won't be tempted as much. Another option would be to bring an extra snack to work that you could eat as you were leaving to go home. This could be a piece of fruit, a sandwich, or a granola bar. This would replenish your glucose levels a little and leave you with more energy to resist temptation and with more energy at home to cook a delicious meal.

Mindless eating

Because so many food choices are made unconsciously, it is very important to be aware of all the food you eat during the day. The TV show *Secret Eaters* makes people write down everything they eat through out the week. While they write down what they think they eat, they're followed with cameras to see what they're actually eating over the span of a week. I've seen people who thought they ate around 1800 kcal a day learn that they were actually eating over 4000 kcal. One guy made lasagna with an entire block of cheese and wondered how he could possibly gain weight. I wondered if they were underreporting on purpose or if the show was set up to make the results extra dramatic, but it seemed like they honestly had no idea they were eating that much.

In the nutrition research community it's generally accepted that a lot of people underreport their food intake. For some groups this can even occur in as much as 70% of people[15]. A lot of this has to do with mindless or unconscious eating. It's fairly easy to down a large bag of chips while you're watching a movie, but if you were to tell someone to count every chip he ate, and thereby make him aware of how much he ate, he would probably eat way less. Eating while you're distracted is one of the best ways to ensure you overeat. Try eating an entire bag of chips while sitting alone in a room with no entertainment versus while you're watching a movie. The movie setting distracts you enough to ignore the satiation signals coming from your body. More on this in Chapter 4.

Mindful eating

I personally don't like the term mindfulness. I like what it stands for, being aware of what you do and not just going through the motions, but the people who generally talk about it are way too hippie for my taste. I personally prefer 'belly full eating', but mindful eating does have its purpose. Snacking unconsciously is a terrible foe when trying to lose weight. Just having snacks within reach makes people eat them more, even when they're not hungry. When candy was kept in a drawer instead of on the desk, people ate 1/3 less[16]. Paying more attention to what you eat can help in a number of ways:

- You enjoy your food more. If someone else cooked for you, try to figure out what she put in the food (and don't forget to compliment her, or at least acknowledge her efforts if the taste is a little off).
- Chewing slower and tasting more of your food leads to more satiation. We'll cover the processes behind this in Chapter 4.
- If you do this with junk food, you'll notice how awful it actually is. The only real way to gorge all that food down is to switch your brain off.

Change your mind

'Progress is impossible without change, and those who cannot change their mind cannot change anything.'
-George Bernard Shaw

To change the way you look, you have to change the way you think. This may sound corny and copied straight from a Tumblr post, but there is truth to it. Tony Robbins, in his bestselling book *Awaken the Giant Within*[17], goes into great detail about how to change your life by changing your mind. He explains thoroughly how your life is formed by your thoughts, beliefs, decisions and actions.

One of his main points is that the first thing that has to change is how you think about yourself, or the stories you tell yourself. If you have been overweight for most of your life, everybody around you knows you as 'the overweight person', and you probably also know yourself as the overweight person. You may have even come to terms with it, making jokes about your own weight even if it is just to make sure other people don't. To change your weight, you have to be able to change the way you view yourself.

Our brains like to be congruent and consistent with their beliefs and convictions. I saw a great example of this on a TV show a few years ago. They showed random men three pictures of different women and asked which of the women they thought was the most beautiful. Once the men had chosen one woman, the men would be distracted and the show's host would quickly switch the picture the man had chosen for a different one and then ask the man why he had chosen this woman. The majority of the men went on to describe why they thought the woman in the picture was beautiful, and in their minds they tried very hard to convince themselves they had chosen this picture. Only a handful noticed the swap and saw that this was in fact not the woman they had picked. What this means for weight loss is that you have a mental picture of yourself as being fat, and everybody around you does as well, which engrains it even further.

To change your weight you have to change the way you think about your weight. In the film *The Secret* they talk about the law of attraction and how you can make things happen just by envisioning them and wanting them bad enough. Through this method you could get a Ferrari by very clearly picturing yourself driving a Ferrari each day. I personally think it's missing a major factor for achieving your goals: effort and hard work, but the principle does have some practical application. Your brain finds it difficult to distinguish between something you picture in your mind and reality.

A somewhat related phenomenon occurs when people try on the new 3D Oculus Rift headset[18]. People are shown a first-person view of a rollercoaster ride. They obviously know that what they're seeing isn't real, but people still get nauseous or fall over when the rollercoaster dives down. Your slow system knows it isn't real, but your fast system finds it very hard to distinguish between an image and reality.

If you can create a very clear picture in your mind in which you see yourself with the body you wish to achieve, your mind will steer your behaviour in a direction that supports that outcome. Also, if you can picture your life with your ideal body, you may be more motivated and more willing to put in hard work. You become more open to opportunities; you become your own *self-fulfilling prophecy*. Arnold Schwarzenegger said he saw himself win a hundred times in his mind before he attempted something. Wayne Rooney visualises scoring a goal to make sure his body knows what to do[19].

What I find just as important as envisioning yourself succeeding is the ability to let go of your old or current self. I don't mean this in the new age hippie sense, that you should let go of your earthly desires and become one with the universe while flying on the unicorn of love. I mean that you have built up your life through years of experiences and events, and all these things combined have caused you to hold certain beliefs and ideas about who you are and why you do things. Most of these beliefs are subconscious, and you rarely stop to think about why you act the way you do, or why you think a certain thought. Fun little experiment: write down everything that pops into your head for five minutes without filtering, hesitation, judging or condemning yourself. You'll be surprised what's going on in that head of yours.

Throughout the years you've formed ideas about your body, food and your health, and these may or may not actually aid you in the process of becoming a better, healthier person. I, for example, held the belief that eating fat was bad and would make me fat for quite some time. When I started learning more about food, I realised I was completely wrong, as we'll discuss in the next chapter, and I let go of that old belief because I realised it was not supporting me. You may have heard in the media that sugar will kill you, or meat will certainly give you stage three cancer within 24 hours of consuming it. These ideas can actually do you harm if you decide to eat no meat at all and develop a nutritional deficiency.

I think half of the progress can be made by learning and receiving better, more truthful information to educate yourself on the things that influence your life. The other half is being able to accept that some of the views you currently hold are not correct and don't support you. This is the trickier part in my experience, because we really love being right and most people deny even the slightest possibility that they could hold an untruthful belief.

This requires an open mindset to learn and consider new ideas. Carol Dweck makes the distinction between a fixed mindset and a growth mindset in her book *Mindset: The New Psychology of Success*[20]. A fixed mindset is one that is well, fixed. To the person with a fixed mindset, the current situation will always remain the same, and there is no chance of improvement. He's basically beaten before he even started. Someone with a growth mindset sees room for improvement, so he isn't stuck in his current circumstances. People with growth mindsets see opportunities, whereas people with fixed mindsets see limits.

The use of emotion for change

Emotion is powerful. The elephant that is our fast system is an emotional beast, and it's much easier for the rider to make the elephant change direction if the elephant wants to do so. Dieting can be quite the emotional rollercoaster, especially if you fail. People are usually quite optimistic when they start a diet. They are full of hope and convinced they'll make a change. Most diets initially work because they restrict calories in some way, although some charlatans claim to have special fruits or herbs that balance your hormones and cause you to lose weight. But the weight loss often plateaus after a while, which decreases motivation, which decreases weight loss and they soon find themselves quitting the diet.

Emotion can be an useful tool when you want to make any change. A sudden emotional burst can be a powerful kick in the butt. It's suddenly much easier to lose weight when you've just heard your current lifestyle will kill you in three months than it is when there is no sense of urgency. It's also much easier to stop smoking once you've heard you're developing lung cancer. Sudden, dramatic events can help people turn their lives around in an instant.

The struggle is that we usually know we should do something, but when there is no sense of urgency, we tend to put things off and pile up the responsibilities for later. This unfortunately seems to be our natural inclination. Our elephants like to relax now and work later. Slowly nudging our elephants in the direction we want seems to be the best option. A fight between the two will just result in a tired rider. This is why we start with gradual changes in our lifestyles instead of trying to disrupt our entire systems.

Emotional eating:
Some people eat because of their feelings. This is often the result of mistaking emotional cues for feelings of hunger. If there are underlying psychological issues that cause you to overeat, just changing your habits most likely won't be enough. In that case it's better to get professional help. Reaching out and asking for help is a sign of strength, not weakness. I try to ask for help as much as possible.
If your problems are less severe, following the steps laid out in this chapter should be enough to make a change.

Chapter summary:
- There are three steps to a habit: the trigger, the behaviour and the reward.
- Breaking habits takes time and effort.
- Habits are not always what you think they are.
- Be aware while you're eating, and don't eat mindlessly.
- Your mind likes to be consistent. Use this to change the way you look at yourself.
- Your mind has trouble distinguishing what's going on in your head from reality, so visualise and become your own self fulfilling prophecy.
- Adopt a growth mindset, and don't be afraid of new ideas.

4. Nutrition 101

You've seen how you can change your behaviour, but another important part of the weight loss puzzle is understanding what you eat. We'll start off with the very basics and work our way up to some more advanced nutrition behaviours.

Our food is comprised of three basic macronutrients: carbs, fat and protein. Then there are two special energy carriers: fiber and alcohol. Carbs and protein both have 4 calories per gram, fat has 9 and alcohol has 7.

Carbohydrates

Carbs are a notorious subject this decade, but they are actually quite helpful once you understand them. Carbs are made up of chains of sugars. The starch in a potato is just long strings of sugars, and the same goes for pastas, rice, bread and any other carb rich food. Sugar is generally known as table sugar, but 'sugar' is actually the name of a group of different substances. The most important sugars are: glucose, fructose and galactose.

Glucose is present is most everyday carb rich foods (pasta, potatoes, rice). Fructose is naturally found in fruit, and galactose is found in dairy. Different foods have different compositions of sugars. Simple table sugar has just one glucose molecule, which means it doesn't have to be broken down, and it can be absorbed very easily. Your body can only absorb single sugar molecules, so longer chains of glucose, commonly referred to as starch, have to be broken down into smaller bits before they can be absorbed, meaning it takes longer to digest them. Think of it as trying to stuff a brick wall through a mailbox. It won't work unless you first disconnect all the pieces and put them through one by one.

Single sugar:

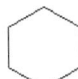

Starch:

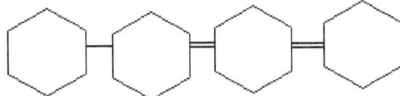

When you're exercising, or moving your muscles in general, you use glucose as a source of energy. The glucose that you digest and take up in the intestine is transported via your blood to your muscles, where it is stored as glycogen in your muscles or in your liver. When your glycogen stores are full and there is still excess glucose in your blood, the rest is either used for heat, energy (e.g. in the brain) or it is stored as body fat.

Fiber

Fiber is special because it is also a starch, but the sugar molecules cannot be separated by the enzymes in the intestine. This means that fiber cannot be absorbed like the other carbs, and it just travels though the body remaining mostly intact. If a normal starch is a brick wall, you could consider this a reinforced wall.

There are two main types of fiber: insoluble and soluble fiber. Soluble fibers dissolve in water, and these fibers are associated with protecting against heart disease and diabetes by lowering blood sugar and blood cholesterol. These fibers are commonly found in legumes, citrus fruits, oats and barley. Insoluble fibers do not dissolve in water, and they are associated with improved bowel movement and alleviating constipation. These fibers can be found in whole grains and vegetables. It is recommended that adults get in around 25-30g of fiber per day. This is quite easy if you eat mostly whole grain sources and enough vegetables and fruit.

Glycemic index, glycemic load

There are people who treat the glycemic index as their bible and will only eat foods that score low on this index. The glycemic index shows how much and how quickly certain foods spike our blood sugar. Pure sugar, or glucose, is used as a baseline and scores a 100. An apple, for example, scores a 36, a banana scores a 51, a boiled potato 78. For more info just search 'glycemic index' on Google Images.

Because it is also important to take into account how much of a food you eat, the glycemic load was developed. This takes the amount of food that is usually eaten into consideration, a banana (120g portion size) scores a 12, a boiled potato (200g portion size) scores a 27.

Now don't freak out and never eat potatoes again - they're amazing for satiation, as we'll discover in Chapter 5. High glycemic foods aren't evil and don't have to be avoided at all costs. I personally would avoid pure glucose because it has no micronutrients or fiber, but let me explain why this glycemic index isn't all that it's made out to be.

Our bodies are digesting food 24/7. Even if you're so hungry you feel like gnawing off your own foot, your body is probably still digesting some food. Your intestine is around 7 metres long, or 24 feet, and while your food passes through this giant tube, it is broken down and small parts are absorbed into your blood. When you ingest food, some of it is broken down in your mouth and stomach and the rest in the intestine.

Most of the food that's broken down gets taken up in the first part of the intestine, called the small intestine. This means you get a peak in uptake fairly soon after you eat. Because your food doesn't stay in the small intestine for days on end, it has to pass through the rest as well. But here's the problem when it comes to testing foods to see how they rank on the glycemic index. To make the tests accurate, the participants hadn't eaten for a long time, and they only ingested one specific food at a time. In real life you rarely wait that long to eat anything, and it's even more rare to eat only one source of carbs without any fat or protein. If you eat a meal with some fat, fiber and protein, those two nutrients decrease the blood glucose spike. Also, if you still have fat, fiber and protein hanging around in your stomach or small intestine from previous meals, they also dampen the blood glucose response. When you pick your carb sources, focus on the amount of micronutrients and fiber they pack instead of the glycemic index.

Fats

Some quick myth busting: eating fat does not make you fat, an excess of calories does. Fat is needed for many processes in your body, like helping your body absorb fat soluble vitamins, hormone production and regulating inflammation. It is absolutely essential to have enough fat in your diet. It's not even optional - your body needs fat. Eating fat is also essential for making sure you get in enough omega 3s, in which most of us are deficient. Omega 3s are found in things like fatty fish (like salmon or herring) and walnuts. There are many more sources, just search 'omega 3 sources' on Google and you'll get hundreds of lists. Omega 3 fatty acids are very important for your brain, and there are also signs that omega 3s have benefits for your heart health[21].

Fat is your main source of energy during rest, and it is also the most easily storable form of energy. Because of its high calorie content (9kcal/gram), it's your body's preferred way to store energy when there's energy left over from a meal. When there is need for energy, fat can be broken down to glucose. This process is not very efficient, so your body will first use your glycogen stores when there is an immediate need for glucose, for example during exercise. If you've ever gone for a run and 'hit the wall' after a while, this is your body running out of glycogen and starting to burn fat as its main energy source.

Structure

Fats are somewhat similar to carbs because they also consist of chains. But fat chains are made up of fatty acids instead of sugars. Fat chains can be saturated or unsaturated. 'Unsaturated' may sound abstract, but it simply means there is a slight bend in the fatty acid chain. There can also be multiple bends in the chain, which we call a polyunsaturated chain. Saturated fat is found in animal products, and unsaturated fats are present in plant based foods, like olive oil. A crude rule of thumb is that unsaturated fat is liquid at room temperature, while saturated fat is solid (there are exceptions, though.)

Saturated fatty acid chain:

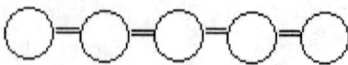

Unsaturated fatty acid chain:

Cholesterol, saturated fat and heart disease

Heart disease or cardiovascular disease (CVD) is the number one cause of deaths globally[22]. Saturated fat and cholesterol have always been notoriously linked to CVD, but that was research from the 1950s combined with a refusal to look at the data presented by more recent and more properly executed studies.

Cholesterol

The mainstream idea about cholesterol is that the cholesterol in your blood is a risk for CVD, and that cholesterol from your food affects the cholesterol in your blood. We're going to debunk this myth in under five minutes.

When you talk about cholesterol, it's useful to distinguish between HDL cholesterol (the "bad cholesterol") and LDL (the "good cholesterol"). Your body gets around 25% of its cholesterol from food, and the other 75% is produced by your liver. When you eat more cholesterol, your liver produces less to keep your total cholesterol in check. So this means that cholesterol from your food doesn't raise your blood cholesterol sky high, because there is a well-equipped system in place to prevent that.

In 75% of the population, cholesterol from your food has very little to no effect on your blood cholesterol levels. In 25% of the population, called 'hyper responders', dietary cholesterol increases both LDL and HDL levels in the blood, but this doesn't affect the balance between the two or increase the risk of heart disease. So in other words: healthy, active people can safely eat two egg yolks a day, which also happens to be packed to the brim with nutrients.

Saturated fat
Saturated fat has been a hot topic for many years because of the supposed link to heart disease. While it's still being debated, recent studies show more and more evidence to support that saturated fat is not a risk factor for heart disease[23]. Being overweight DOES play a major role in all kinds of diseases. It is possible that overweight people eat more saturated fat, so there is a correlation, but it does not mean saturated fat causes heart disease.

Although there is no clear concensus that cholesterol and saturated fat are bad for your health, there is still no need to go nuts and consume 100g of saturated fat a day. Generally speaking, it's pretty safe to follow the intake guidelines set by the World Health Organisation. They recommend a maximum of 20g of saturated fat for women and 30g for men. From the data I've seen, there is no harm in going over that, and I sometimes do, but too much of anything will have negative effects.

Trans fat, f*ck that

There is one type of fat that should be avoided: trans fats. These factory made fats are mostly present in commercial baked goods and refined snacks like cookies, ready to serve pies, chips and most things that go in a frying pan. Trans fats mess up the balance between the HDL and LDL cholesterols, which has some serious negative side effects. Some countries are working on banning trans fats, but there is still a way to go before your food is trans fat free. Trans fats may also be labeled as hydrogenated fat.

Protein

Protein is my personal favorite. It keeps you satiated the longest, helps you grow and keeps you strong. Protein, like carbs and fat, is built from strings of smaller building blocks. These blocks are amino acids, and there are around 20 different ones. There is a distinction between essential and non-essential amino acids. Non-essential amino acids can be produced by our bodies, while essential amino acids are the ones the human body cannot produce on its own, which means we have to get them from our diets.

Protein can come from either animal or plant sources. Animal protein is generally considered more complete because it contains all of the amino acids. Most plant based proteins lack a few amino acids, and these should then be consumed from different sources. There are a few plant based proteins with more complete amino acid profiles, like quinoa or soy.

Protein is involved in a number of processes, including:
- Building materials for your muscles, skin and even blood
- As hormones
- Transporters - you may have heard of hemoglobin, which transports oxygen from your lungs to every part of your body.
- Enzymes - the proteins you ingest from your food are actually broken down by other proteins called enzymes.

One amino acid:

Protein:

Alcohol
Alcohol is not considered a nutrient because it does not support health, quite the opposite in fact, but it does contain kcal. The problem with acohol is not just the amount of kcal you consume (a beer can easily pack 100+ kcal), but it also has a few other effects:

- As we all know, alcohol tends to cause disinhibition (or a shut down of the brain's slow system), and this mostly results in after party munching on everything that your brain finds delicious, like anything deep fried, kebabs, and pizza.
- Alcohol disrupts the metabolism of fat and causes your body to store more of the fat you eat.
- Alcohol makes you lazier, especially if you're hung over the day after. The intention to work out can easily be overrun by the urge to sleep and watch Netflix.

Party people advice:
Alcohol is a big part of most of our cultures, and there is no need to abstain completely to achieve a healthy, good looking body. I recommend you try to eat a protein and fiber rich meal before drinking heavily to keep off the munchies somewhat. Another idea is to have a nice, pre-cooked, healthy meal waiting for you when you get home. Try to avoid stuffing down massive amounts of fatty foods, as you are more likely to store it as body fat.

If you are tracking your kcal (as we'll discuss later in this chapter) try to always be in a kcal deficit when you are drinking, because your body has more difficulty storing carbs as fat when you are in a kcal deficit.

That's nice and all, but how much should I eat of each macronutrient?

First, you have to calculate how much kcal you need per day to maintain your current weight. This can be done by Googling: 'freedieting kcal calculator'. There are many more ways to calculate your kcal need, but this one seems to be fairly accurate. Once you fill in your stats, it shows you how much kcal you have to eat to maintain your weight. Ignore the 'fat loss' and 'extreme fat loss' numbers. This maintenance number is a rough estimate, because everyone is a little different when it comes to calories. You can check if this number is correct by doing the following experiment.

Track your kcals with an app like Fatsecret or Myfitnesspal for a few weeks and start out by eating the calculated number of maintenance kcals. Now, if this number actually is your true maintenance level, then your weight should stay the same. If your weight goes up over the course of those weeks, you are eating above your maintenance level, and your actual maintenance level is lower than the calculated one. Vice versa if you lose weight, then your maintenance level is actually higher.

Once you have determined your maintenance kcals, you can start to play around with that number to meet your specific goal of weight loss or weight gain. If you want to lose weight, some recommend that you should eat 500-1000 kcals less than your maintenance. I have an issue with this statement. It doesn't take into account that people can vary enormously in size and kcal needs. A small woman who needs 1500 kcals and a large man who needs 4000kcals have very different results if they both drop 1000kcals. The woman will nearly starve, and the man, although he will probably be hungry, can still eat a large amount of food.

I prefer to take your maintenance kcals and multiply them by .8 to .9, depending on how fast you want to lose weight. For the woman this would be 1200-1350kcals, for the man 3200 to 3600. It is possible to drop your kcals more drastically to lose fat faster, but as you read in the first chapter, fat that is lost quickly has a good chance of coming back quickly.

To gain weight (for people who work out hard and want to become more muscular), I like a surplus of 200-500kcals. It takes some experimentation to see what works for you, because your maintenance also shifts slightly when you gain more muscle mass. Start out with a surplus of 200kcals, and see if your weight changes over the course of two weeks. Depending on your goals, you can then alter the surplus to get the results you want. A surplus that is too high will result in too much fat gain, so start slow and keep a close eye on your weight.

Now that you have your desired kcal number, start filling it up with carbs, protein and fat. I can't tell you the perfect way to divide your kcals over your macronutrients, but consider the following a rough example:

- Carbs: 45-65% of your total kcals
- Fat: 20-35% of your total kcals
- Protein: 10-35% of your total kcals

Carbs and protein have 4 kcals/gram and fat has 9 kcal/gram, so with these guidelines it is quite easy to calculate what your intake should look like.
This all sounds great in theory, but in practice there is no real need to stress about these numbers. The most important parts are:

1. Get enough protein, so no less than 10% of your total kcals should come from protein.
2. Get enough fat, so no less than 20% of your total kcals should come from fat.

Once you have met both of these needs, you can play around, and there is no need to adhere to any strict number unless you like having strict rules for yourself.
So let's try this in an example. Let's say I need 2500kcals. I might want to eat 80g of fat for the day, which amounts to 720kcals. Next I would like 150g of protein, which gives me 600kcals. Then I have 2500 minus 720, minus 600 = 1180kcals left to fill with carbohydrates. 1180/4= 295g of carbs. Et voila, you have mastered macronutrient tracking.

All this may seem a tad overwhelming, and you probably don't feel like doing math when you want to eat, but just take the info with you and we'll apply this knowledge in Chapter 6.

Micronutrients
Besides the macronutrients, there are the all-important micronutrients. Micronutrients are vitamins and minerals that help with all kinds of processes in our bodies. Vitamin D and calcium support strong bones, vitamin A keeps our eyes healthy, zinc helps our hormone production and much more. Don't let the 'micro' part fool you. Without these essential little helpers, our bodies are weaker and more vulnerable to diseases. Vitamin A deficiency can cause blindness, vitamin C deficiency can cause scurvy and vitamin D deficiency can cause low bone density.

There is a lot to be said about vitamins and minerals, but I will try to keep this section as comprehensive as possible. For more information on vitamins and minerals, like how much you need of each vitamin or mineral, just look up that specific vitamin on Google.

If you eat plenty of varied meals with enough vegetables and fruits, you're not very likely to have any serious micronutrient deficiencies. There are a few occasions on which you have to pay a little more attention:
-    Your body produces a large part of its own vitamin D during the summer through exposure from the sun. But during winter, the sun hours decrease and we're usually more covered up, which means we produce less vitamin D. In this

case it's smart to supplement with some vitamin D pills or something like cod liver oil.

- Pregnant women require extra folate. This is quite common knowledge, but not knowing this can lead to serious birth defects.
- Certain diets or lifestyle choices can lead to deficiencies, for example not eating meat puts you at more risk of a deficiency of vitamin D, B12, calcium, iron and zinc. Protein intake should also be monitored.

Processed foods

The problem with processed foods isn't that they're toxic because of the E-numbers. For non EU people: E numbers are substances that are strictly tested for safety and are found to be safe for human consumption at doses comparable to normal intake. The 'E' stands for European. My issue with E-numbers is that nobody knows what happens if you ingest 50 different ones per day, and what effect they have all together. So I recommend, just to be safe, that you mainly eat foods that are non-processed and E–number free. The other concern with processed foods is that they are ridiculously low in micronutrients and fiber. When your main ingredient is high fructose corn syrup (candy, pie, cookies) or white flour (pizza) it's hard to make the entire thing nutritious. This means you're more likely to develop a nutritional deficiency, and this is, in my opinion, the more serious problem of the two.

Dairy

In many countries (including the Netherlands) kids are brought up with tons of dairy. The main reason dairy is supposed to be good for you is because it has a lot of calcium to support strong bones. The funny thing is that research has not shown that calcium supplementation alone is associated with a decrease in the risk of fractures[24].

There is evidence that calcium, especially in combination with vitamin D supplementation, does help to prevent bone loss, but this effect is very minimal[25]. There is also a difference in quality of the dairy depending on where in the world you buy it. Most of Europe has strict laws concerning the use of growth hormones for cows (as in, they don't allow it), but the US is a bit more lax with this subject. Dairy is fine if you know it comes from a good source and your body tolerates lactose. I would prefer yoghurt over milk, this is more of a personal preference than science, although yoghurt does have nice bacteria that are good for your intestines.

What foods to eat

When it comes to picking exactly what foods you should eat, common sense is your best friend. Less processed foods are generally better than processed foods, and fresh is better than old. Many products today have claims on them like, '30% less fat', 'no added sugar', or 'rich in protein'. The fact that these products need those health claims in order to be seen as 'healthy' says a lot. When you walk through the vegetable and fruit aisle in the supermarket, you rarely see any of these claims, because fruits and veggies don't need any claims to give them the image of being healthy.

Some people are very concerned with the amount of sugar in fruit. Although it is true that plain sugar isn't your most healthy option, fruit also has fiber and many vitamins and minerals that far outweigh the negatives. Most people don't even meet their daily recommendations of two servings of fruit each day, so worrying about the amount of sugar is trivial.

My personal eating regimen is built around the 80/20 principle. I eat 'healthy' foods 80% of the time and the 20% is open for things like birthday cake and snacks. You already know that restrictive dieting works poorly (remember the polar bear experiment?), so trying to eliminate all bad foods will most likely backfire. With the 80/20 principle, you avoid this by having a clear agreement with yourself that you eat well most of the time, and when you're offered a piece of cake at a birthday party, you're free to eat it.

'Healthy food' is very subjective and depends upon what your body needs and where your personal health lies. I consider brown rice to be healthy, but if you only eat brown rice for a year, you'll definitely get some serious health issues. To keep things simple, use common sense when it comes to healthy eating.

Some examples of healthy foods:

Beans, brown rice, (sweet) potatoes, smaller fish*, unprocessed meat, pretty much all fruits and veggies, whole grain products.

Some examples of unhealthy foods:

Most processed foods, fries, chips, cookies, pretty much anything with low fiber combined with high amounts of fat and sugar.

*There are a lot of pollutants in the ocean, and over time, these get stored in fish. Every time one fish eats another fish, the built-up pollutants are also ingested and stored. Small fish (like mackerel, sardines, herring and salmon) only eat a few other fish, so it builds up only a low level of pollutants. Bigger fish like tuna eat tons of other fish, and they store all those pollutants from the fish they eat, so they have high levels of pollutants. Most store-bought tuna shouldn't be eaten frequently because of the high levels of mercury.

Chapter summary:

- Carbs, protein and fat are all built up from smaller building blocks and have to be broken down before they can be digested.
- Carbs are fine, but look for good fiber content and try to go easy on the sugar most of the time.
- Fat doesn't make you fat; your body needs it. Cholesterol and saturated fat aren't the devil, but don't go crazy with them. Avoid trans fat.
- Protein is awesome.
- Alcohol makes you hungrier and makes you store more fat. It can be fun though, so if you drink try to eat protein rich foods and low fat.
- When it comes to macronutrient ratios, getting in enough protein and fat are the basics. If you meet that criteria the rest doesn't matter as much.
- Dairy is fine if it comes from a good source and your body tolerates lactose.
- If you eat well 80% of the time, you can afford a snack here and there.
- Use common sense.
- Eat mostly non-processed foods, because those contain more micronutrients and fiber.

5. Understanding Your Body

The King and Queen of Weight Management: Satiation and Satiety

Satiation and satiety are often used interchangeably when referring to the feeling of fullness after a meal, but they do mean slightly different things. Satiation refers to the point during a meal when you feel full and stop eating. Satiety is the period you keep feeling full until you want to eat again and enjoy your next meal.

When losing weight you're looking for good satiation combined with long satiety. Many people eat to the point at which they feel very full or stuffed. The goal of a meal should never be to feel full to the point that you have to lay down to keep yourself from exploding. **The goal is to not feel hungry after your meal**. The problem with satiation is that it takes a while to kick in. You can down a ton of food and only later realise you ate way too much. We'll talk about how to combat this down below.

Satiation is dependent on mostly the sensory qualities of the food or meal, like the meal size, how good it tastes, or if it is a solid food or a liquid.

Satiety is mostly dependent on the nutritional qualities of the food, like the number of kcals, amount of fiber, and amount of protein.

There is an order to how much the macronutrients satiate you. Protein is the best satiater, then carbs and then fat. At the very bottom is alcohol, which can make you even hungrier. Fiber is amazing for satiety because of its water attracting properties - it literally fills you up. So any meal with a good deal of fiber and protein will keep you feeling full for quite some time.

Sugar

Sugar, on the other hand, is one of the main nutritional reasons so many people today are overweight. Sugar has 4 kcal/gram like any other carb, but the problem is that when you drink something like a soft drink with a ton of sugar, it barely satiates you, if at all. To make matters worse, pure sugar causes a big spike in blood sugar, which in itself isn't the end of the world, but when your blood sugar comes back down it dips a little lower than baseline.

Low blood sugar causes your body to want to eat again because it senses a lack of blood sugar that has to be replenished.

When you normally eat a decent sized meal, your blood sugar gradually increases and gradually comes back down to baseline, and you then get hungry again. But during this time you are satiated and you have no desire to eat much food. What sugar does is mess the system up and cause you to want to eat again very soon. Because there is also no protein or fiber, there is little to no satiation and you remain hungry.

There are a few satiation tricks to support your weight loss:

1. Balanced meals with fat, protein and carbs cause less of a blood sugar spike and keep you satiated longer.

2. Fat causes your stomach to empty less frequently and this too keeps you fuller longer.

3. Avoid sugary snacks when you want to keep the weight off; they don't fill you up and can make you even hungrier.

4. Liquid meals satiate less than solid meals do. The exact mechanisms are still being debated, but it may be because chewing and the feeling of solid food in your mouth tells your brain you're eating. Your brain needs to have enough stimulation from chewing and moving food around in your mouth to achieve satiation. When you drink something like a sugar sweetened beverage, this system is bypassed and your brain doesn't register it as eating. Zijlstra and colleagues tested this in a study in which they found that the ad libitum (non restricted, eat as much as you comfortably want) intake was 30% more for the liquid version of a product than for the semi solid version[26].

5. Water soluble fibers have been shown to improve satiety and decrease the amount of food eaten at the next meal, compared to low fiber meals.

6. Zijlstra and colleagues have also done research on the effect of bite sizes and the speed of eating on total intake. They gave volunteers either 5 or 15-gram pieces of chocolate every 3 or 9 seconds (sorry chocolate lovers, they're not taking volunteers anymore).

    They were instructed to eat until they felt comfortably full (ad libitum). The results weren't surprising. The 15-gram piece group had a higher ad libitum intake than the 5-gram group did. The group that got a piece of chocolate every 9 seconds also ate less than the 3-second group, which is in line with the theory that satiation takes a while to set in. Later studies by Bolhuis et al. and Weijzen et al. found that doubling the eating speed increased ad libitum intake by 30%[27,28]. You could put this into practice by, for example, eating with a smaller spoon or fork, taking the time to chew a bite thoroughly, or telling a story during dinner to decrease your eating speed.

7. Distraction is a main culprit in overeating. We are prone to eat more when we don't notice we're eating. This is why you can easily eat an entire bucket of popcorn during a movie, but it would probably be pretty hard or at least less fun to eat it without any distractions. Studies have shown that even the number of people at dinner can increase how much we eat. This is most likely due to the fact that when there are more

people present, we are more likely to pay less attention to our food and more to the people surrounding us, which seems like a normal thing to me.

I'm not saying you should eat alone to lose weight. Please don't - there are way more social and health benefits to spending time with friends or family. That said, it is something to be aware of. When you are going for that second plate, ask yourself if you are truly hungry or if you just want to eat. A good trick is to wait 5-10 minutes before attacking for a second time, this gives your body some time to let the satiation kick in, and you'll probably have less of a need to eat.

8. You're probably familiar with the expression, "My eyes were bigger than my stomach." This expression comes in handy when you're trying to lose weight via the availability bias. The availability bias entails that we tend to get more of what is widely available. For food this means that when you put an enormous amount of food on your plate, you tend to eat more than you would if the portion were smaller. This also means you will probably be just as satisfied by putting a smaller portion of food on your plate and stopping after that. This can also work the other way around with vegetables, if you make a massive salad, you'll eat more than you would if you had made a smaller serving.

Satiety Index

The satiety index tells you how satiating a food is compared to white bread, which is set at 100 as a baseline. White bread is quite bad at satiating due to its low amount of fiber and protein, so 100 isn't really an achievement. They measure the amount of satiation by giving a 240 kcal portion of a food to a group of volunteers and then measuring how much they eat at the next meal. Cake and doughnuts come in at a whopping 65 and 68, and a Mars candy bar doesn't do much better with a 70.

Fruits tend to do pretty well, with oranges scoring a 209, apples 197 and bananas 118. Anything with a decent amount of fiber also scores pretty high, like oatmeal 209, brown pasta 188, baked beans 168 and whole wheat bread 157. High protein items score high as well: eggs score a 150, beef 176 and ling fish 225.

Some surprising findings include popcorn, which scores a 154. This could be because you have to eat a pretty large serving of popcorn to get to 240 kcal (assuming you don't add butter or sugar). Boiled potatoes score a ridiculous 323, making them the king of satiating foods. Baked potatoes will most likely score a little lower because of the added fat to bake them, but they're still nice.

This list isn't perfect. Jelly beans, for example, scored a 118. This could be because 240kcal of jelly beans made the volunteers a little nauseous.

Overall, the most important factors are:

- The water content of the food, making the food bulkier and heavier
- The fiber and protein content.
- The size of the food. One of the reasons potatoes satiate so well is because you need to eat a large amount to get a decent amount of calories.

Inside versus outside eating stimulus

A baby knows when it's hungry, and soon after the baby finds out, so does everybody within a hundred metre radius. Internal signals tell a baby when to start crying for food and also when it has had enough. It's pretty hard to find an overweight, breast fed baby. When we get older we tend to rely more on outside signals, like a clock, or when we get home from work to tell us when to start eating. An experiment from the sixties put a clock in a room and then asked overweight and non-overweight people to fill in a bunch of forms[29].

The researchers made sure there were plenty of snacks in the room, and the participants could eat freely. What the participants didn't know was that the clock had been tampered with, and this provided some unusual results. Overweight people ate more than the rest when the clock had been set ahead, because the clock said it was close to dinner time and they should be getting hungry by now. Instead of paying attention to the signals coming from inside their bodies, they relied on outside signals to determine when and how much they ate. This is also where dieting fails. When someone is on a diet, he is told to ignore the signals coming from his body, like hunger. Instead of listening to your body, you are to trust some one-size-fits-all diet to make you lose weight.

The fat loss/ fat gain cycles
Fat loss or fat gain isn't a linear process that just keeps on going in one direction. Throughout the day you gain and lose fat. Yes, you can gain and lose fat in the same day. In fact, you don't have much of a choice. After each meal your body goes **anabolic** (from the greek 'anabole' = to build up) and digests the food. It can, for example, use the carbs to convert to glycogen, use the protein to help repair your muscles and use the fat for energy. But there is an amount of kcal left that can't be used directly. These kcals are stored for later as fat. Later in the day, when you haven't eaten for a while and your body is going **catabolic** (from the greek 'katabole' = to throw/break down), it starts breaking down the stored fat and glycogen to use for energy.

Weight fluctuations

Fat loss can be a tricky fellow when it comes to measuring accurately day by day or even by a scale at all. Our bodies consist of around 60% water, which means that a 70kg person (or 155lbs) is 42kg (or 93lbs) of water. This amount tends to fluctuate with the amount of water you drink, the amount of salt you eat and the amount of carbs you eat. I've done an experiment in which I lost 5kg or 11 pounds in 2 days just by reducing how much water I drank and lowering my carb and salt intake.

My body fat barely changed (if any at all), although I did look leaner because I was holding less water. This can be a deceiving first boost when you start any low carb diet, because you usually lose quite a bit of weight during the first week, which feels great, but after that the weight loss slows down tremendously, causing some people to quit the diet because they don't see the same progress. To provide the extra kick while you're down, you gain all that water weight right back once you start eating your normal amount of carbs and salt again.

Small psychology side note: One reason people quit after not seeing the same progress is because of the 'contrast bias'. Let's say one person has 10 bucks and the other has 5 bucks. If we take 2 dollars from the first person and give 1 dollar to the second, the first person will have 8 bucks and the other will have 6. What's funny about our brains is that we would be happier in the shoes of person 2, even though the first person still has more money. This is because we get a rush of good feelings when we improve, but we feel worse if we lose things. This is another reason we go for gradual and steady weight loss, which keeps us feeling good because we improve every time.

Fat loss shouldn't be thought of as a 'I'll be skinnier the next day' process, although it is the result of our day-to-day activities as you'll see in the next chapter. It's more healthy and mentally relaxing to look at the general direction your weight is going over a period of weeks or months. A lot of people freak out when they step on the scale and they've gained 3 pounds compared to the day before. This is nonsense by the way. It is incredibly hard to gain even 500g or one pound of fat in a day (trust me, I've tried).

Chapter summary:

- The goal of a meal is not to feel stuffed, the goal is to not feel hungry.
- Sugar doesn't satiate.
- Eat slower, chew more, smaller bites and portions.
- Satiation takes some time to kick in, so don't rush to that second plate.
- Balanced meals are best.
- Listen to your body, not outside stimuli.
- You lose and gain fat constantly.
- Your weight fluctuates greatly due to water and glycogen.
- Look at fat loss as a journey, not a race.

6. Lifestyle and Exercise

The best way to lose weight is not to hop on a diet, because we know now that diets often stop working the moment you quit the diet. What you should do is make gradual changes in your habits and behaviours so you can maintain your health and weight with the smallest amount of effort. Think about brushing your teeth. It's not something you have to put any effort into because it's a habit and you're used to it. This is because you have built a pattern and because of that, you don't really have any feeling toward brushing your teeth. It's **just something you do.** In this chapter we'll cover how you can optimize your lifestyle to support creating better habits and making your life that much more awesome.

Exercise

Exercise is considered weight loss' golden boy, and it obviously has enormous health benefits that reach far beyond just maintaining a healthy weight. But when it comes to pure weight loss, there is something that most people overlook. Before we delve into that, I would like to explain a few concepts so we can dive in prepared. Losing weight happens via a kcal deficit: you eat less than you burn. You could just eat less than your maintenance amount of calories and lose weight that way. Another way is to exercise more, burn more calories than you eat, and create a deficit that way.

Let's say person A and B both need 2000kcal to maintain their weights. Person A eats 1800kcal, and creates a 200kcal deficit that way, which means the total deficit at the end of the week is 7 x 200 = 1400kcal. Person B decides to keep her food intake the same, but instead starts working out three times a week and burns 500kcal per workout. The total deficit at the end of the week here is 3 x 500 = 1500kcal. Both ways create roughly the same deficit, and both person A and B lose weight.

What is missing in this picture is the fact that exercise is not the only way to burn calories.

Energy expenditure; the good, the bad and the lazy

Our energy expenditure, or the kcals we burn, go into four different pools. At the bottom is your basal metabolic rate or BMR. The BMR is what your body burns in order to just stay alive when you lie completely still. This accounts for roughly 50-65% of your energy expenditure. Next is the thermic effect of food or TEF, which means the energy it costs your body to break down the food you eat. Your intestines have to work pretty hard to digest all those proteins, carbs and fats, and all of this costs energy. Your TEF accounts for roughly 10% of your total energy expenditure.

You might have seen people who like to pray on the uninformed and try to sell them diet plans that will boost their metabolisms by 679% (or any other ridiculous number) with some special food. What most of these diets do is recommend more protein. Because protein has the highest thermic effect, it takes the most energy to break down. Although I like eating protein, the extra kcals that are burned to digest the protein are not something to write home about. I recommend you focus your efforts on more useful things than trying to raise your metabolism, like improving your habits or increasing your NEAT. It also happens to be way easier and more helpful for weight loss to increase your NEAT than it is to increase your metabolic rate.

NEAT stands for non-exercise activity thermogenesis, or in common words, the amount of kcals burned by things like walking the dog, vacuuming, writing, tapping your foot, showering and maintaining your posture, anything that isn't considered exercise and isn't taxing on your body. NEAT accounts for around 10-25% of your energy expenditure. This number varies a lot because your NEAT can be increased without too much effort and increases the kcals you burn in a day quite drastically.

Exercise accounts for a much smaller part of the total energy expenditure than NEAT. Exercising is made out to be the eighth world wonder for weight loss, but NEAT accounts for almost double the amount of energy expenditure, and that's pretty neat*. Increasing your NEAT is a very easy way to increase the kcals you burn throughout the day.
*had to be done.

Exercise, especially resistance training like lifting weights, has a ton of benefits like increasing your bone density (which lowers the risk of bone fractures for the rest of your life), making you look good in a swimsuit, building discipline and confidence by seeing yourself improve, and much more. Therefore I highly recommend you do some form of intense exercise, mostly just because it's fun, but because you'll also get all the benefits mentioned above.

Seven ways to increase your NEAT:

1. Take the stairs instead of the elevator.
2. Is the car really necessary for that 5-minute ride? Pop in some headphones with an audiobook or your favorite music and walk or cycle there.
3. Clean the house a bit more often. A clean house doesn't just feel good mentally, but half an hour of cleaning can burn quite a few calories.
4. Take walks frequently. This not only clears your head but also helps clear out your fat reserves.
5. Try to stand instead of sitting for long periods of time. You can try switching it up and do half an hour each at a time. I've noticed I get much more work done if I take short breaks from sitting every half hour. It gets you out of your pattern, and when you get back to your work you're way more productive.
6. If you can't stand while you're working, get a DeskCycle, or some other type of small hometrainer. It's a small pedal station that fits under your desk, and you can pedal comfortably while you're working.
7. An even better option is to get a treadmill desk. This sounds weird, and it kind of is, but it's also pretty cool. It's just what the name says, a treadmill with a desk on top. Sitting for long hours is one of the main reasons so many people don't get enough daily movement in. A desk like this does cost a pretty penny, but the saved expenses on medical bills should balance that out

nicely. It is meant to be put at a speed that is even lower than normal walking so you don't really sweat and even stuff like typing is still very doable.

Feel free to add your own twists to things to make them work for you specifically. You probably have way more ideas than I could come up with. If you have kids or a dog, you could take them to the park more often. They'll love it and get some more exercise themselves. We're looking for overall life improvement; a healthy lifestyle doesn't have to be taxing or boring.
The main point with NEAT is that little things add up. Try to implement some of these things and you'll be amazed at how much difference small things can make. Don't try to do all these things at once or you'll burn yourself out. Pick one that you think will work best for you and implement that into your daily routine. Once you've done that, come back and pick another. We're aiming for small, gradual changes in lifestyle, not a sprint ending in a crash.

Cooking
Cooking is a bit like art: most people like the result, but few care to do it themselves. Cooking can be either great or a disaster, depending on who you ask. Home cooking can be an amazing tool for losing weight because you know exactly what you're putting in and that allows you to make very healthy, delicious meals. The downside is that cooking usually takes a lot of time, and in today's busy world time is not something we have in excess. One solution to this is batch cooking.

I like to cook something like rice, couscous, pasta or bulgur in bulk. Then all I have to do is make some type of sauce or topping and I've got myself a meal. An expansion on this idea is to dedicate one evening to cooking food for the entire week. You could for example cook pasta, rice and couscous and then make three different sauces and throw all of that in the freezer (separately, of course). When it's time to eat, you just grab one of the sauces and some pasta, couscous or rice and you throw that in a pan to heat up, maybe add some extra spices and you've got yourself a meal.

This 'preparation principle' can be applied to almost anything. If you like to take sandwiches to work for lunch, you can make all your sandwiches for the entire week in one evening and put all of them in the freezer. Then all you have to do is take one sandwich out in the morning, and by the time lunch time rolls around it's ready to eat. Most foods don't really taste much different after freezing and defrosting (as long as they're sealed in air tight containers), although I recommend you add fresh vegetables instead of freezing them. This will make your dish ten times better.

A less aggressive alternative to batch cooking is to just cook too much. This will give you extra meals without much more time invested.

Get creative with this and find what meals and ingredients you like.

How to make cooking much more fun:

1. Get a good set of knives. The two most frustrating things when cooking are: burning something and having a dull knife. You can get some pretty good knife sets for under 50 bucks, and it's definitely worth the investment. I really like the Victorinox 3 ¼ inch paring knife for my smaller stuff. It works wonders for cutting tomatoes.
2. Try local farmer's markets. Farmer's markets are usually cheaper than supermarkets and way fresher. They also often carry some items you don't often see in a supermarket, like fresh sauerkraut, passion fruit or exotic peppers.
3. Seasonal veggies and fruits are often way more delicious than when they're out of season. So try some seasonal items; they might just surprise you with how good they are.
4. Invest in a few cookbooks or some type of cooking course to up your cooking game. Cooking is so much more fun when you have some basic knowledge about how to prepare certain ingredients. Youtube also has thousands of videos on how to prepare pretty much anything.

Chapter summary:

- Aim for gradual changes over time.
- Exercise is awesome, but NEAT is also important.
- Look for ways to improve your NEAT and activities that fit into your life.
- Cooking is great for your health. Make it fun and use batch cooking to save time.

7. Getting started

'A good plan violently executed now is better than a
perfect plan next week.'
-George S. Patton

It takes roughly 66 days to replace a habit, and I'm not
going to lie, it is tough. For practical purposes, it makes
sense to prioritize the bad habits that are now affecting
you the most and focus on those first. Focus and
willpower are required to consciously change the habits
that are not supporting you right now, but the key is to
save that precious willpower for the most essential
moments.

For example, it's a good idea to eat a big meal before
going to do the groceries for the coming week. This way
you have sufficient glucose ready to make all kinds of
decisions and you don't go into a supermarket hungry,
which is a lost battle. Make that willpower work where it
counts. Don't be penny wise and dollar foolish; exert
your effort on the big decisions.

Getting to know your food

'What gets measured gets managed.'
– Peter Drucker

We've discussed tracking kcals in Chapter 3, but the goal
is to improve your healthy eating and lifestyle habits to
make tracking and other tools unnecessary. But as you
know, it takes a while to change habits, and to start this
off it's very useful to get a clearer understanding of the
foods you're eating.

Once you eat mainly healthy foods with lots of fiber and enough protein, it will actually be harder to gain weight than to lose weight, just because you won't be hungry enough to eat those extra calories. Weight gain usually happens when you eat too many cookies, pizzas, doughnuts, candies and other non-satiating junk.

I've tracked my kcal for about six months, and although I don't think six months is even necessary, I can now eat whatever I like and I don't gain weight unless I want to. I eat plenty of brown rice, oats, salads, pasta, fish, meat and my fair share of pizza now and then, but my weight remains the same. This is what I would like you to experience: a guilt-free, stress-free relationship with food.

For the first few weeks on this journey I'd like you to track your kcals with an app like Fatsecret or Myfitnesspal. This takes less effort than most people think. Once you're used to the app, it'll only cost you around three minutes a day, and that's a pretty good investment if it results in having a grip on your food intake. This period is mostly meant to make you more aware of what is in the food you eat and how much you're eating of it. We are terrible at estimating how many calories are in certain foods, especially when it comes to larger portions. Even nutritionists have this issue, so weighing and tracking your food intake is a great way to prevent underestimation. An especially tricky category is the food with labels that contain claims like '30% less fat' or 'contains no trans fats'.

Weighing your food may seem ridiculous, and I think it definitely is if you do it all your life. Once you've measured your food for a while, especially things you eat more often, you'll know what one serving of rice looks like.

If you think the scale is a tad much and there is no way in hell you're carrying a mini food scale with you everywhere you go (with things like batch cooking you can weigh your food at home and make your life a bit easier), using serving size cups for which you already know the measurements can come in handy.

Once you start eating healthier and you keep doing this for a while, you'll start to crave junk food less frequently, in part because you know how it makes you feel. I feel great when I eat healthy, but if I gorge on junk food one evening, I definitely pay the price the next day. My energy is lower, I have the occasional headache, and I have more trouble focusing.

Tracking your weight

You already know that your weight fluctuates because of the water and glycogen you hold, so some people recommend you only measure your weight once a week to get a more accurate portrayal of your progress. This is not true. A study found that people who weighed themselves every day found it easier to control their weight[30]. They indulged in binge eating less often and then were less depressed about their daily meeting with the scale. Measuring yourself carefully and often makes it easier to detect deviations and it gives you more insight to see if what you're doing is working. There are even scales that track your weight for you[31].

Tracking your movement

As human beings we are designed to move, not to sit in a chair for 10+ hours a day. Measuring your activity increases the chances of succeeding, and there are tools to help you do exactly that. A pedometer (apps like WalkLogger) measure the amount of steps you take during the day. Most experts recommend 10000 steps a day. This might sound like a ridiculous number, but you'll see that little walks add up quickly. When I'm having a busy day that involves a lot of work at a desk, I take around 3500 steps. These days happen once in a while and that's fine, but most days I try to put in some extra effort and walk to the grocery store or go for a walk in the park. When I do something extra like that it's easy to get upwards of 7500 steps. I'm definitely not perfect. I average at around 6000, but perfect is not the goal. Find what you need for your life and what amount of activity makes it easy for you to stay in shape.

Exercise

You should do some form of exercise, period. There are just too many mental and physical benefits that come from exercise to allow yourself not to. Some might not be too happy with that news, others have zero issues with it because they are already active. Below we'll explore some exercise options so everyone can reap the benefits from becoming fit.

But, I have no time

I've heard the excuse: 'But I don't have time to exercise' dozens of times.

'When somebody says: 'I don't have time….., simply add 'for that'. You have the same 24 hours as everybody else, decide how to spend it.'
-Jason Capital

If you have time to watch TV or Netflix, you have time to exercise. Working out two times a week only has to cost you 2 hours. You probably spend more time than that mindlessly checking your phone. I do think it's important to be able to rest and take a break, but many people spend too much time on the wrong things. Seneca in his book *On the Shortness of Life*[32] says that people are very greedy when it comes to their money and property, but they readily waste their time like it means nothing to them. Don't play the victim of the circumstances you created. You have plenty of time to exercise, but you may have to give up some less useful activities.

The gym

If you don't want to hit the gym for any reason, that's fine, but don't knock it till you try it. Most people I know (including myself) felt a little out of place in the gym the first few months, and that, combined with the fact that you'll probably have no idea what you're doing, can be a turn off. To prevent this I recommend you find someone who has been going to the gym for a while who can take you under her wing and show you the way. A personal trainer is also a great way to motivate yourself, because once you've paid for the service and scheduled a session, you'll think twice about skipping a workout. A third option is to find a buddy with whom to conquer the gym. Frodo would be nowhere without his Sam, and a gym buddy will motivate you to keep going even if you've already given up five times.

A great, simple weight lifting program is *Jason Blaha's 5x5*. Just type that into Google and you'll find a video explaining the entire program. I also recommend getting a good personal trainer to work on your technique for a few weeks when you decide to start working out. There are a lot of bad trainers out there, though, so preferably get someone with good credentials.

Another idea is to search the exercise you want to try on Youtube. There are hundreds of videos explaining how to properly perform that exercise.

Quick gym etiquette to make sure you don't make a fool of yourself:

1. Place a towel on the machine you're using and wipe any remaining sweat once you're done.
2. It isn't necessary to chat with everybody if you don't want to, but you'll probably build a circle of familiar faces or even friendships over time.
3. If you don't want to be disturbed during your workout, just put in some headphones, and 95% of people will get the message.
4. Ladies, it's a gym, not a party, so please don't wear layers of make up and an outfit that covers 10% of your body.
5. Guys, wearing a tanktop is fine, but no one likes to see a guy's nips slip out during an exercise, so please pick something that fits.
6. Asking other people for help is encouraged and can be quite flattering for them. This gives them the opportunity to be your Mister Miyagi, just make sure you don't ask them while they're in the middle of doing an exercise.

Quick side note for the ladies: lifting weights does not make you the hulk. Some women have this idea that they may gain 30 pounds of muscle after a workout and look hideous. I can assure you that most men struggle to gain muscle mass, and women are way less inclined to get big, so lifting weight does not make you muscular instantly. It also takes years to gain a significant amount of muscle, even for guys, so you won't wake up one day and be huge all of the sudden. What lifting weights does is make your legs and butt toned and curved in a good way (I think all the men can agree on this). Running doesn't build a bikini body, squats and lunges do. It's also nearly impossible for a woman to get big and super ripped without steroids. Those pictures of uber muscular woman are almost always the result of steroid use.

A team sport

If you know you prefer to play on a team, see what local clubs there are in your neighbourhood and reach out to ask if you can try a free class; 99% of the time they'd love to have you. This can be exciting, but for the more shy people reaching out to an entirely new club may be a bit intimidating. Shyness is definitely a breakable habit, but for now, ask friends or family what sports they're playing and go along for a class with them if you find a sport that seems fun to you. A team is a great thing because human beings are designed to be in groups that work together. This makes us feel like we are part of something, and that is a great thing. Also, once you are part of a team you have an obligation to show up and play your part in the team.

Home workouts

Thanks to the internet and a few enthusiastic personal trainers, there are thousands of videos and programs available that show you what you can do to exercise from your home. This is super convenient and I work out at home sometimes when I don't feel like going to the gym but still want to move a little. Just Google 'home workout', and you'll immediately be immersed in tons of options, so pick one that you like and you can start right away. Preferably get one that isn't just an ab routine. Look for squats, lunges, pull ups, and push ups, to make sure you get yourself a more serious workout.

Some type of class

Classes are great for the same reason as team sports. They add a layer of commitment that is outside yourself. You can also go with friends, which is especially helpful in the beginning. Check Google for local classes and see if there is something that suits you.

Strategies for a successful change in habits

First, you must focus your efforts on the habit that is holding you back the most right now. For some this might be not exercising enough, for some it might be smoking, for others eating too much junk food. Since you started reading this book you probably already have an idea of what habits are your biggest downfalls. If you really don't know what habit to tackle first, ask friends or family what they think will help you the most. They often see things that might not be obvious to you.

When you've got a habit narrowed down, go through the habit breaking steps mentioned in Chapter 2.

Identify the triggers, remove them as much as possible and replace the old habit with a better one.

This may sound easy, but it can be quite difficult, especially once you're past the 'this is new and exciting' phase. Your mind likes new stuff, but once something is old news, the excitement usually fades. To keep yourself on track, here are a few tips to ensure you follow through. Some of these things might seem simple or unnecessary, but I've noticed that the people who actually do these have a way higher chance of success.

Set realistic goals

A good starting point is to look in the mirror, take a 'before' photo, weigh yourself, and then create a feasible plan of attack. Most people mess this up and set ridiculous expectations for themselves. People did this so frequently that the British bookie, William Hill, took bets in which people could predict how much weight they were going to lose and in what period of time. It seems foolish to accept such a bet; the dieter can not only determine the terms, but also the outcome. Although the rewards could reach up to five thousand euro, the dieters still lost the bet 80% of the time. It's better to aim lower than you'd like to and meet or even exceed your weekly/monthly goals than it is to fail your own expectations. The average bet at William Hill's office was 1,5kg (3 pounds) of weight loss a week for a total of 35kg (77 pounds).

Sites like stickK.com or fatbet.net do a similar thing as William Hill. StickK.com lets people decide their own goals and punishments, but the success rate of people at stickK is way higher than the people who placed their bets with Mr. Hill. This is because stickK doesn't accept any bets higher than one kilo (2,2 pounds) of weight loss per week for a total of 18,5% of their body weight. Again, slow and steady wins the race.

Understand what you are doing to yourself

It helps to very clearly define what exactly you'll miss out on if you do not change your old destructive habits. If you are currently overweight and below 60, this could be not being able to see your grand children grow up. Write these things down and keep them at the back of your mind. It is okay if you get a bit depressed doing this, but don't sob and feel like the victim. Take control and use it as motivation to accomplish what needs to be done. Visualize what aspects of your life will change for the better if you complete the process of making better habits. I had a bad habit of procrastinating a while back.

My list to stop my procrastinating contained things like: 'I have so much more free time and less stress because I have my work done way in advance. This allows me to travel and see more of the world'. Try to write these things as if you are currently experiencing them, instead of 'I will'. This again comes down to the consistency bias: once you have the mental image in place of yourself succeeding, the actual success is much more likely to happen. Put this list in a place where you look at it frequently, like on the fridge, on your desk or next to a mirror. Your willpower will often diminish, so little boosts like these at the right moment make all the difference.

Is writing things down actually necessary? Yes, it is. David Kohl, a professor at Virginia Tech, found that people who write their goals are nine times more likely to accomplish them. Yes, nine freaking times more likely to reach their goals. What he also found is that only 10% of people actually do it and only 1% review their goals regularly. That 1% probably consists of the most successful people around. So write down your goals, and preferably check on them regularly. Don't get depressed (and possibly eat away your feelings) if you didn't accomplish your goals, look at the results like a scientist. A scientist doesn't get mad at the results he got from a study, he analyzes them and looks to find out what caused them.

Your goals aren't the only things you should be writing down. Jason Selk, author of the book *10 Minute Toughness*, says that your products (the goals) as well as your process (how you're going to get there) should be clearly written down. This could look something like this: 'End goal: lose 40 pounds. Process: Walk 5000 steps a day, join the volleyball team and practice twice a week'. John Wooden, one of the most famous basketball coaches of all time, was asked once what he focused on during a game. What he said might surprise you: He looks if his guys are running in a straight line or in a banana pattern. When he was asked why he didn't pay attention to the score or the opponents strategy, he explained it very simply: The shortest distance between two points is a straight line, so if his guys run in a straight line instead of a banana pattern, they will always be a little bit faster. This is what will show up on the scoreboard.

Solely focusing on the product isn't the best strategy. Focusing on the process of getting there and making sure that part is perfect automatically leads you to the product. See the big picture, but do the little things right. To assist you with this, make a calendar with daily, weekly and monthly goals with boxes that you can tick off. Despite the fact that it just feels good to tick off boxes, it gives you a sense of accomplishment and pride to be able to cross out everything you've already accomplished. Accomplishing the goals you set out for yourself also gives you a lot of trust in yourself, which is a great side benefit.

Gary Keller wrote a great book about achieving your goals titled *The One Thing*[33]. It's an awesome book on it's own, but the extras he provides on his website **www.the1thing.com** provide a lot of additional value. If you go to: **www.the1thing.com/resources/tools-and-forms**, you'll see the '66-day calender' and 'Your long-term goals' files. Downloading those and printing them out gives you a nice and easy plan.

Make your goals public

Apply the same concept as sites like stickK.com do: share your goals with a friend or family member (or if you're feeling brave, post them on social media) and let there be consequences if you do not accomplish the goals you set. The reason this helps is because now you can't get away with not doing what you have to do without consequences. Make this an official thing and make a simple contract that you and your accomplice sign, this way you allow yourself no excuses. And trust me, your mind will try to make up all kinds of excuses when your willpower runs out. Putting money on the line can definitely help. Losing money feels terrible.

Postpone instead of restricting

Restricting only makes you want it more, and restricting only works as long as your willpower is available. If you're sitting at a buffet and you're constantly trying to resist the urge to get some ice cream, you'll wear yourself out with each attempt and end up giving in at the end. What is strange and hopeful is that saying to yourself, 'I'll have this later', is way less destructive than saying, 'I can't have this'. Nicole Mead and Vanessa Patrick researched this in an experiment in which they designed a setup with a short movie and a bowl of M&Ms[34].

Volunteers were divided into three groups. One group could eat as many M&Ms as they wanted, group two couldn't eat any of the M&Ms, and the third group was told they could have M&Ms later. The first group of course ate more than the second and third group, this was to be expected, but here is where the actual experiment began. The researchers asked the participants to come to another room one by one in which they would fill out another form.

Unexpectedly, a researcher would show up with a bowl of M&Ms and tell the participant that everyone else has already gone home and these are left over. The researcher would then leave again and the volunteer could then eat as many M&Ms as his or her heart desired, because it was unmonitored and it wouldn't matter anymore, or so they thought. Of course, the researchers weighed the bowl before and after they handed it out and could see exactly how much one person had eaten.

Now, you would expect the postponed-pleasure group to attack the bowl, this was of course what they had told themselves was the deal. The surprise was that the postpone group didn't splurge at all, in fact, they ate less than the group that was told they couldn't eat anything. One theory to explain this is that postponing doesn't feel as negative as limiting yourself does. You'll still get the reward, just later. This means you waste less willpower resisting and can focus your energy on things that matter more. Do you remember the polar bear experiments by Daniel Wegner? He also found that postponing a thought allows people to worry less about something.

Have a plan going in

'By failing to prepare, you are preparing to fail.'
-Benjamin Franklin

Let's say you're trying to lose weight and you have been invited to a dinner with friends and family. You know there will be many temptations there, and pure willpower won't be enough to keep you on track. Let me share a few strategies you can try beforehand.

1. Sit next to the small eaters. Human beings are very social creatures, and we have the tendency to conform to the perceived social norm. If everyone around you is done eating after one plate, you'll be less likely to delve in for a second plate than you would be if you sat next to the bottomless pits of the party who go for thirds or even fourths.

2. Another strategy is to have your answer ready when temptations show up. This reduces the need to think and consider, which in turn reduces your need to use mental energy. So before you even go to the party, agree with yourself that when they start serving fries, you'll just say no. Another example, when they come up to you and ask you what you'd like to drink, pick something with zero or minimal calories. These choices then become defaults because you've already decided and you waste no energy having to decide on the spot.

3.   A more drastic approach is to socialize more with people who are skinnier. I'm not saying you should abandon your overweight friends, but social research shows that skinny people and overweight people do tend to form groups[35]. Again, social norms play a major role in our behaviour, so hanging out with fitter people will be better for your weight loss. Just going to a gym or sports club can help with this, as most people there are fit or trying to become more fit, so building a social circle there can assist you.

'One of these days is none of these days.'
-    Unknown

Throughout this book I've bombarded you with knowledge, and it's understandable if you feel a little overwhelmed and already forgot half of it. The goal right now is to pick a few points from this book and start implementing those into your life. It's easy to want to do too much at once and not know where to start. If you want to do too much, you can end up paralyzed by the amount of options, or 'paralysis by analysis'.
A good place to start is to ask yourself what things will have the highest impact. If you're familiar with the Pareto principle you'll know about the 80/20 rule. 80 percent of the results are caused by 20% of the actions. This rule goes for almost any area of life, 20% of the work you do gives you 80% of the results, 20% of the costumers bring in 80% of the revenue.

Don't get caught up on the exact number, that's not the point, it may sometimes be 90/10 or 70/30, but the principle works. Find out what 20% of your actions produce 80% of your results. If you decide to focus on resisting a single piece of candy but at the same time are only getting 100 steps a day, you're not being very efficient with your effort. Leverage your energy, apply it where it counts most.

That said, pick something and start. All this information won't do you any good unless you apply it. You don't need a perfect plan or the exact blueprint laid out in advance. The most important part is to start.

Chapter summary:

- Use your willpower for the big decisions.
- Pick some things from this book and work with those. There is no need to do everything at once.
- Tracking what you eat for a few weeks allows you to learn a lot about your food.
- Measuring yourself frequently helps you stay on track.
- You need to do some form of exercise (and you do have time for it).
- Set realistic goals for yourself.
- Very clearly write down what you'll miss out on if you don't change.
- Write down the process as well as the product goals. Make a plan that incorporates both.
- Make your goals public.
- Postpone eating instead of restricting it.
- Have a plan beforehand.
- Just start. You don't need a perfect plan.

So what are you waiting for? Let's Start.

Thank you for reading this book! I really appreciate your feedback and love to hear what you have to say.

With your input I can make coming books better.

Please leave me a helpful review on Amazon!

Thanks so much!

-Rens

[1] World Health organisation, 2015.
http://www.who.int/mediacentre/factsheets/fs311/en/
, visited at 23-12-15

[2] Alexander, D. D., Weed, D. L., Cushing, C. A., & Lowe, K. A. (2011). Meta-analysis of prospective studies of red meat consumption and colorectal cancer.*European Journal of Cancer Prevention*, *20*(4), 293-307.

[3] Walley, A. J., Asher, J. E., & Froguel, P. (2009). The genetic contribution to non-syndromic human obesity. *Nature Reviews Genetics*, *10*(7), 431-442.

[4] Landecker, H. (2011). Food as exposure: Nutritional epigenetics and the new metabolism. *BioSocieties*, *6*(2), 167-194.

[5] American psychology association, 2015
http://www.apa.org/helpcenter/willpower.aspx?item=1
, visited at 23-12-15

[6] Baumeister, R., & Tierney, J. (2011) *Willpower: Rediscovering the Greatest Human Strength*. New York: Penguin Press.

[7] Tangney, J. P., Baumeister, R. F., & Boone, A. L. (2004). High self-control predicts good adjustment, less pathology, better grades, and interpersonal success. *Journal of personality*, *72*(2), 271-324.

[8] Tangney, J. P., Baumeister, R. F., & Boone, A. L. (2004). High self-control predicts good adjustment, less pathology, better grades, and interpersonal success. *Journal of personality*, *72*(2), 271-324

[9] Haidt, J. (2006). *The happiness hypothesis: Finding modern truth in ancient wisdom*. New York: Basic Books.

[10] Wegner, D. M., Schneider, D. J., Carter, S. R., & White, T. L. (1987). Paradoxical effects of thought suppression. *Journal of personality and social psychology*, *53*(1),

5.

[11] Herman, C. P., & Mack, D. (1975). Restrained and unrestrained eating. *Journal of personality*

[12] Polivy, J. (1976). Perception of calories and regulation of intake in restrained and unrestrained subjects. *Addictive Behaviors, 1*(3), 237-243.

[13] Lally, P., Van Jaarsveld, C. H., Potts, H. W., & Wardle, J. (2010). How are habits formed: Modelling habit formation in the real world. *European Journal of Social Psychology, 40*(6), 998-1009

[14] Duhigg, Charles. (2012) *The power of habit :why we do what we do in life and business* New York : Random House

[15] Macdiarmid, J., & Blundell, J. (1998). Assessing dietary intake: who, what and why of under-reporting. *Nutrition research reviews, 11*(02), 231-253.

[16] Painter, J. E., Wansink, B., & Hieggelke, J. B. (2002). How visibility and convenience influence candy consumption. *Appetite, 38*(3), 237-238.

[17] Robbins, Anthony. (1991) Awaken the giant within. New York: Summit Books

[18]https://www.youtube.com/watch?v=GoQ0OXJCbaE

[19] http://www.theguardian.com/football/2012/may/17/wayne-rooney-visualisation-preparation

[20] Dweck, C. S. (2006). *Mindset: The new psychology of success.* New York: Random House.

[21] Swanson, D., Block, R., & Mousa, S. A. (2012). Omega-3 fatty acids EPA and DHA: health benefits throughout life. *Advances in Nutrition: An International Review Journal, 3*(1), 1-7.

[22] http://www.who.int/mediacentre/factsheets/fs317/en/

[23] Siri-Tarino, P. W., Sun, Q., Hu, F. B., & Krauss, R. M. (2010). Meta-analysis of prospective cohort studies evaluating the association of saturated fat with cardiovascular disease. *The American journal of clinical nutrition*, ajcn-27725.

[24] Bolland, M. J., Leung, W., Tai, V., Bastin, S., Gamble, G. D., Grey, A., & Reid, I. R. (2015). Calcium intake and risk of fracture: systematic review

[25] Tang, B. M., Eslick, G. D., Nowson, C., Smith, C., & Bensoussan, A. (2007). Use of calcium or calcium in combination with vitamin D supplementation to prevent fractures and bone loss in people aged 50 years and older: a meta-analysis. *The Lancet, 370*(9588), 657-666.

[26] Zijlstra, N., Mars, M. D., De Wijk, R. A., Westerterp-Plantenga, M. S., & De Graaf, C. (2008). The effect of viscosity on ad libitum food intake. *International Journal of Obesity, 32*(4), 676-683.

[27] Bolhuis, D. P., Lakemond, C. M., de Wijk, R. A., Luning, P. A., & de Graaf, C. (2011). Both longer oral sensory exposure to and higher intensity of saltiness decrease ad libitum food intake in healthy normal-weight men. *The Journal of nutrition, 141*(12), 2242-2248.

[28] Weijzen, P. L., Smeets, P. A., & de Graaf, C. (2009). Sip size of orangeade: effects on intake and sensory-specific satiation. *British journal of nutrition,102*(07), 1091-1097.

[29] Schachter, S. (1971). Some extraordinary facts about obese humans and rats.*American Psychologist, 26*(2), 129.

[30] Wing, R. R., Tate, D. F., Gorin, A. A., Raynor, H. A., Fava, J. L., & Machan, J. (2007). " STOP regain": Are there negative effects of daily weighing?. *Journal of consulting and clinical psychology, 75*(4), 652.

[31] http://www.amazon.com/Borg-BDM950KD-45-Weight-Tracking-Scale/dp/B00477ISXS

[32] Seneca, Lucius A. *On The Shortness Of Life: Life Is Long Enough If You Know How To Use It.* Trans. C.D. N. Costa. New York: Penguin Group, 1997. Print.

[33] Keller, G., & Papasan, J. (2012). *The one thing: The surprisingly simple truth behind extraordinary results.* Austin, Tex.: Bard Press.

[34] N.L. Mead, V.M. Patrick, 'In praise of putting things off: how postponing consumption pleasures facilitates self-control'

[35] Christakis, N. A., & Fowler, J. H. (2007). The spread of obesity in a large social network over 32 years. *New England journal of medicine, 357*(4), 370-379.